THE DUE DATE

BIRTHING IN THE RIGHT SEASON

Delisha Easley

The Due Date: Birthing in the Right Season.

ISBN: 978-1-7379081-4-2

Imprint: Independently Published.
Publishing Assistance by Reaching While Teaching LLC

Books may be purchased in bulk quantity and/or special sales by contacting the author at info@delishae.com

Book Cover Designed by T. Harty Designs
Edited by Crystal Clear Editing

To book Delisha or inquire about her services, email **info@delishae.com** for more information.

TABLE OF CONTENTS

DEDICATIONS

My Auntie Lessie and Grandma Willie May, you both were matriarchs in our families that truly impacted our lives generationally. You both taught me the importance of staying connected to God and relying on His strength, I miss you both daily. Your prayers are still being answered. Thank you!

Princess Raquel "Rocky" Hudson, my lil sis for life, you taught me to live in the moment. I will continue to live my life of royalty and help others discover their royal priesthood (1 Peter 2:9). As you'd always say, "We aren't spoiled, we are well taken care of " yes, and amen sis. Love you!

My Auntie Nadine AKA "My twin"! Your words live on and I will continue to make you proud by fulfilling all God has called me to do. The world didn't get to cherish your love, wisdom, and kindness, but your daughters and I will make sure they know about it through your words. Love you and thank you for being YOU!

SUPPORTER SHOUTOUTS

Ebony Haliburton

Uncle Gary & Auntie Ramona Holland

Kendra Sims

Margaret Smith-Williams

Shanine Young

Pastor Deloris Ward

Pastor Dexter Easley

Angela McIntosh

Atarah Sevier

Tramaine Brown

Alisha Wilkerson

Dionte Chantel

Sade Jones

Olea Harris & THINNKK Pretty

and many others!

SPECIAL THANKS

Mommy, thank you for being my midwife numerous times and I appreciate you for that. Thank you for showing me the discipline it takes to truly be a living sacrifice in God's Kingdom. Your nurturing ways have developed me into the woman I am today. I thank God for choosing you to be my mommy.

Love you always,

Your Princess Delisha

FOREWORD

I have watched with pride the quest Delisha Easley has been on to walk in the calling God has on her life. Her intellect has served to broaden the expanse of the spiritual knowledge she is gaining.

In The Due Date: Birthing in the Right Season; Delisha uses her intellect and spirituality to approach this most critical subject matter in spiritual development, the need for a midwife. She has been thorough in her research and has combined it with her own life's experiences to present this compelling read.

As you read this book, you are invited by the author to reflect on your own spiritual journey to become more aware of the need for the midwives God provides for us in the various birthing seasons of our lives.

I applaud Delisha for delving into this subject matter and look forward to additional writings from this anointed young woman.

Be prepared for an incredible journey as you explore all that is in store in The Due Date: Birthing in the Right Season.

Blessings,
Elder Mavis V. White

INTRODUCTION

The Due Date is a book that gives an overview of a key person we need in our lives more than we think; a midwife. Guys before you stop reading, hear me out. In the spiritual realm there is neither male or female so we are all able to bring forth what God has placed within us. Throughout the book, the role of a midwife is examined and displays the necessity of everyone having one or multiple throughout their birthing seasons.

Many people reading this probably successfully brought forth "babies" without a spiritual midwife and that was great. However, with this next "baby" you need the wisdom, guidance, and prayers of a midwife. Books have used the story of Mary and Elizabeth focusing on someone else's baby can make yours leap. I'd like to venture deeper and say: can you show me how to carry and deliver what everyone doubted could ever happen come through you? An important thing to remember is that your spiritual midwife is only with you for a season. It may be a total of a year but the functioning of a midwife doesn't usually exceed that. Also, if they were your midwife once doesn't mean they'll be it again. Every pregnancy is different so you may need a more seasoned midwife for your first pregnancy, while at your fourth or fifth you can get someone a bit newer.

The goal of this book is not to make you feel good, but rather wake your soul up to the necessity of what your spirit needs to bring forth. Galatians 5:17 (NIV) For the flesh desires what is contrary to the Spirit, and the Spirit what is contrary to the flesh. They are in conflict with each other, so that you are not to do whatever you want. Our flesh is looking for an emotional reaction but our spirit is here to obey the things of God. You aren't going to "feel" like getting up at 3am to pray this dream, vision, calling or assignment through. You aren't going to "feel" like fasting during the holidays, if that's what it takes. We want to pray like Jesus in Luke 22:42, but real talk, we do want our will to be done, because it's easier. However, when you decide to take the cup and take up your cross, it's time to go to work. The time for contemplating if God "called" you is over; it's time to walk in the authority He has given you. As Jesus needed the donkey in Luke 19:31, the Spirit is saying to you now, "I have need of you." Believe that and go do all He has told you.

CHAPTER 1

First in the natural then the spiritual

Midwives are beginning to be called upon often again for various reasons. However, before moving forward with this book it's vital to know what a midwife is. The first definition is what the natural role of a midwife is.

Midwife-- a person trained to assist women in childbirth.

Spiritual midwife-- a person trained to bring forth the promise God has placed in you.

Before moving forward there are a few things I'd like to clarify when reading this book. The perspective is from a spiritual standpoint. There aren't necessarily prerequisites to reading this book, but there are some foundational things that need to be understood. In Galatians 3:28 it states, "There is neither Jew nor Greek, there is neither slave nor free, there is neither male nor female; for you are all one in Christ Jesus."

Therefore, as you continue to read this book, know it's for anyone that needs to bring forth what's spiritually in them into this natural world. Also, I will describe things that are natural first to help the readers receive the revelation of spiritual understanding.

A midwife has numerous responsibilities that happen before, during, and after pregnancy.

Responsibilities of a midwife

Certified midwives have many specific responsibilities as part of their work including:

- Primary care for expecting mothers and women
- Diagnosing and treating patients
- Providing references to specialists
- Collaborative work with physicians

- STD testing and treatment on expecting parents
- Education and preparation for new parents
- Handling labor and delivery
- Care for newborns during the first 28 days of life
- Assisting during cesarean sections
- Emotional support for expecting mothers
- Prenatal examinations
- Postnatal examinations
- Training to deal with complications that may arise during labor and delivery
- Prescribing medicine to patients
- Advanced practice training with physicians
- Overall health evaluation

The responsibilities of a spiritual midwife as part of their assignment are:

- Provides primary care for the individual, (care is the provision of what is necessary for the health, welfare, maintenance, and protection of someone or something.) Take a moment to think about whether anyone in your life at this moment is genuinely concerned about your welfare. Did you come up with at least one person? If not, this may be a good time to re-evaluate your circle of family and friends.
- Diagnosis (the identification of the nature of an illness or other problem by examination of the symptoms) and treat (deal with in a certain way.)
- Collaborative with The Great Physician (Jesus, Mark 2:17) praying specifically concerning you and your "baby".
- Handling labor and delivery (Isa 37:3) This is an area I will elaborate on further, but I like to reference the verse in Isaiah

37:3 "This day is a day of distress, rebuke, and rejection; for children have come to birth, and there is no strength to deliver." A very real thing that can happen in delivery is a baby being ready to come out and a mother unfortunately not having enough strength to push the baby forth. In the natural, it is called FTP (failure to progress), and if this happens, various techniques, medicines and/or cesarean delivery is the only option to ensure the safety of mom and baby. However, if the extended period of time with progression continues the mother and baby both may be injured. Let's go a little deeper into what these extended periods of time can look like for mother and baby. The mother could have additional complications such as severe hemorrhaging, in which a hysterectomy is performed. A hysterectomy not only causes the mother the inability to bear children in the future, but also triggers premature menopause. Unpacking this in a spiritual sense, when you don't have the strength to push forth what God has given you and man's assistant/tools are used the increase in having a safe delivery are jeopardized. We often say it's in God's hands but still rely on the plans of man alone. We are open to consequences of our actions not only endangering ourselves, but our baby and possible future babies. It's not enough to conceive the promise but we must also ask God to give us the ability to deliver full term what He has promised, with His strength. The promises God has placed in us are often impossible to man and therefore will take supernatural strength and great faith to bring forth. Which is why the next responsibility of the midwife is essential.

- Emotional support (Luke 1:26-45)-- this area is essential in pregnancy as your emotions can be all over the place, but getting support from someone who is going through or been down a similar path is just different. In the first chapter of Luke, Mary is told by the angel Gabriel that she will bring forth the son of God, but Mary was a virgin and not married to her fiancé just yet. The miraculous was coming and she was chosen because of Joseph's lineage to King David and her purity. Meanwhile, her older cousin Elizabeth was also in the midst of a miraculous pregnancy, as she and her husband John were past "conception" years. However, we know God works in the "impossible." Who better to support Mary through this than her cousin Elizabeth? Elizabeth was six months pregnant at the time so she had some time on this pregnancy path and could be a great resource and support. In verse 36, the angel Gabriel references Elizabeth's miraculous pregnancy to somewhat encourage Mary that it's possible. Mary goes to visit Elizabeth after this encounter. Upon the greeting of Mary, Elizabeth's baby (John) leaped in her womb and Elizabeth was filled with the Holy Spirit (Luke 1:41). We've often heard commentaries and sermons in regards to Elizabeth's baby leaping, but not as much on the fact that she was filled with the Holy Spirit. This entire encounter is simply amazing. Both women had miraculous pregnancies and became more connected because of the assignment placed on their babies. One baby preparing the way for the next to become the Savior of the world. Simply Wow! A great takeaway from this story is to find someone filled with the Holy Spirit that can make your baby leap. Elizabeth and Mary encouraged each other. Remember emotional support is needed at all stages of your pregnancy, delivery, and after.

- Training to deal with complications in labor and delivery (Rom. 8:18-25, 30, 2 Cor. 12:8-10, Ps 8:2-- "Out of the mouth of babes and nursing infants you have ordained strength, because of your enemies, that you may silence the enemy and the avenger.") The definition of complication is a circumstance that complicates something; a difficulty, an act of complicating elements or things. Something that introduces, usually unexpectedly, a problem, or change. Labor and delivery is difficult enough, but adding complications jeopardizes the survival of you and the child. When complications are happening while we are trying to bring forth, the verse in Romans 8:18 comes to mind: "...that the sufferings of this present time are not worthy to be compared with the glory which shall be revealed in us." The glory is all worth it. You will be like the woman in labor who is sorrowful but when she has given birth to the child, she no longer remembers the anguish (John 16:21). Some of you are in labor and almost about to deliver, but too focused on the current anguish to even fathom that you won't remember because the joy from the birth of your child will outweigh it. I'm your assistant midwife begging you to focus, breathe, and PUSH! A complication may come but you have a community trained to deal with these complications. During this time it's not about being strong, but rather trusting what you know God promised. The promises of God are yes and amen, meaning it is so and it will be established (John 7:38). No matter how painful it may be, how long it's taking, how hard it is to push or if complications arise, just remember if God promised it then you will bring it forth! Labor and delivery is where many people give up without realizing each pregnancy is different, and though this one may seem more difficult than others, it doesn't mean it won't happen. As I'm writing this book many complications tried to hinder it from coming forth at the right time. Oftentimes when a mother is unable to push they have to do a C-section, which makes for more possible complications. For some of you, the baby is coming no matter what. Either you need to pull on your strength or prepare for surgery. We are living in a time that all God has placed in you is wanting to come out and needs to be on this earth for such a time as this. We have to be as Esther–willing to die for this (Esther 4:14-16).

- Care for newborns in the first 28 days of life-- (28 can mean balance and the word Lamb,) According to Luke 1:56, Mary remained at Elizabeth's house for 3 months, Mary not only saw the parallels of her cousin's pregnancy but helped her bring forth. The scripture does not go into detail how Mary served or what she gained for staying an additional three months. I would like to assume that Mary was learning a lot about motherhood and preparing for her own journey. This is why it is vital to have sisters supporting us along the journey. Oftentimes God places individuals in your life on similar journeys to help you along yours. Keep moving.

These responsibilities are upheld with the greatest level of dedication and commitment. A midwife becomes a member of the family because of the responsibilities and duties entailed in the entire process. The midwife stays in constant communication and check-ups for a month and half, sometimes longer to ensure the mom and baby are fine. This is very important as postpartum can begin as early as a few days after birth or a year. Now for physician and hospital births you are only a number of many giving birth and quickly released from care; then it's left up to you to schedule an appointment after the first six weeks.

A spiritual midwife is giving the proper care for the mom and baby throughout the birthing process. Having a spiritual midwife in this day and age is beneficial to the health and fully developed promise within you to come forth. Now let's go into why we each need a spiritual midwife.

HEART QUESTIONS: What's the difference between spending time with God and isolation? How has your isolation hindered you from bringing forth?

CHAPTER 2

Why do you need a midwife?

Here I'd like to take a moment to explain the difference between a doula and midwife. Midwives have medical training and/or experience. The medical training is not just a few courses; they have to enroll in a two-three year post-secondary education training, which has to be taken at an accredited midwifery school approved by the Medical Board. [1]

A reason everyone can't become midwives is because just like in the natural world, it takes extra work. A spiritual midwife also needs post-secondary educational training. Your Dean or Head Instructor is the Holy Spirit. In John 14:26, it says the Holy Spirit will teach you all things and I like how the NIV states, "...and will remind you of everything I (Jesus) have said to you." As an educator, I'm the first one to encourage someone to receive more education to gain knowledge, but we must remember only applied knowledge is powerful.

The late great Mother Boyd would often say, "Make sure you pass the course or you'll have to repeat it." In spiritual education you have to work to pass courses as well. However, in this journey the Head Instructor is also your Tutor! Referring back to John 14:26, Jesus said the Holy Spirit would remind you of everything. That alone gives me the confidence to push through until graduation.

A midwife is specifically brought into your life to help you prepare to give birth. Every birth is unique and sacred. The necessity of a midwife is that they can go beyond what's seen in the natural world. Not only can they identify an area of improvement or hindrance, but they know how to get you properly fit for birth.

---

[1] (in California footnote https://www.mbc.ca.gov/Licensing/Licensed-Midwives/apply/)

Having someone pray with you concerning a matter is one thing, but to have someone toil or tarry with you until the promise is birthed, that's unique and rare. Midwives in the natural or spirit are rarely called upon anymore for various reasons. However, I believe God has called some intercessors to rise up and be a midwife to help these next generational leaders bring forth all God has placed in them. Everyone's role is not to have the microphone. Honestly, I'd rather have God's ear than man's mic.

The old saying, it takes a village to raise a child is very true. It takes a village to nurture the promise God has given you. As mentioned before, a midwife does not take away from any mentorship, coaching, or support you're receiving from anywhere else. A spiritual midwife is an individual that is focused on you and taking your concerns before the Lord.

So, why do you need one? Right now you may have a feeling inside of you that this specific project, book, ministry, or actual child is supposed to come forth through you. However, you keep delaying the delivery.

You must not delay any longer! There is a blessing in bringing forth at the right time. This chapter opened with the verse Isaiah 37:3b (NKJV), for the children have come to birth, but there is no strength to bring them forth. What God has promised is coming forth, but do you have the strength to bring forth? In the spirit there is no epidural.

Studying the birthing process I discovered there are complications in premature birth, as well as prolonged births. The timing of God's promise is just as important as the promise itself.

Before moving on to the determination of the due date, let's define what a doula is.

Doula is a trained companion who is not a healthcare professional that supports a pregnant woman during labor. Consider a doula as a peer mentor or close friend. They are quite supportive but not qualified to help assist you in the birthing process.

The due date for God's promises also takes time but can always speed things up (Exodus 1:19). We must prepare to bring forth when the okay from God has been solidified.

Due dates in the natural world are estimates that can change, but when labor begins nothing is changing the baby coming forth.

In the natural there are three stages of labor:

First stage is when your contractions increase, and your cervix begins to dilate (the longest stage).

Second stage is when your cervix is fully open. This is the part where the baby moves through the birthing canal by pushing with your contractions.

Third stage is after the birth of your baby, when your womb contracts and causes the placenta to come out.

While reading, I pray you received the revelation of where you may be in the labor process. However, there may be a few of you reading saying, "I'm not sure labor has come yet." Below are a few early signs of labor.

Giving birth - early signs of labor

- your waters breaking (rupture of the membranes);
- backache, or an upset stomach;
- cramping or tightening, similar to period pain;

- a feeling of pressure, as the baby's head moves into the pelvis;
- an urge to go to the toilet caused by your baby's head pressing in your bowel.

If you are experiencing pressure in various aspects of your life, you may be in labor. Being in labor is a good thing, because it's a reminder that the baby is coming soon.

"Whenever a woman is in labor she has pain, because her hour has come; but when she gives birth to the child, she no longer remembers the anguish because of the joy that a child has been born into the world." John 16:21

Your hour has come for you to bring forth. Therefore, be ok with the discomfort, pain, aches, urges, and cramping– the promise (baby) is coming soon. After the birth, the joy that the child brings outweighs the memories of the pain.

No matter what's happened in the past concerning other promises, it is now time to truly bring forth and deliver what God has placed in you. Many of the promises we are bringing forth aren't for us. Remember Hannah– she believed God for years for a child; and when she finally conceived and gave birth, she rededicated him back to the Lord. Only seeing him once a year (Ref. 1 Sam 1:9-28 NLT).

I will share more about that story later, in regards to having the ability to give the promise back to God, but for now let's just highlight her dedication to serving the Lord and pleading for her heart's desire for years.

In the New Testament we see a similar story with Elizabeth, mother of John the Baptist. Elizabeth and her husband Zacharias were up in age to be conceiving, but it was the will of God. What if we were told that today? Would we have enough faith to handle the news? At this point, the great story of Abraham and Sarah was well known, so God doing a miracle similar to this had been done before, but it was so long ago. However, maybe this is why Elizabeth was okay with it and Zacharias had a more difficult time. That scenario is even more ironic considering Zacharias was a priest who studied the scriptures of old. The story goes on to explain that Zacharias' prayer for his wife to have a child was coming to pass (Luke 1:13). God is about to answer some prayers you may have forgotten you've prayed.

In verses 13-17, the angel Gabriel gives a detailed explanation of how much joy they will have and who the child will become in the future.

"But the angel said to him, "Do not be afraid, Zacharias, for your prayer is heard; and your wife Elizabeth will bear you a son, and you shall call his name John. And you will have joy and gladness, and many will rejoice at his birth. For he will be great in the sight of the Lord, and shall drink neither wine nor strong drink. He will also be filled with the Holy Spirit, even from his mother's womb. And he will turn many of the children of Israel to the Lord their God. He will also go before Him in the spirit and power of Elijah, 'to turn the hearts of the fathers to the children,' and the disobedient to the wisdom of the just, to make ready a people prepared for the Lord." (Luke 1:13-17 NKJV)

As a parent, this can give you numerous emotions of excitement, nervousness, fear, and happiness. However, there is no room for doubt. Even though Zacharias had prayed for a child for years, and an angel is literally having a conversation about his future son, the fear that came upon him in verse 12 blinded him from all the angel had just said.

And in verse 18 Zacharias replies, "How shall I know this? For I am an old man, and my wife is well advanced in years."

When God is answering a prayer request we have to not question "how" He's doing it. For years I've struggled with not trying to figure out how the promises of God concerning my life are coming to fruition. If we focus on the "how" and "why" we get distracted from the promise. The "how" in this story caused Zacharias to become mute for nine months (Luke 1:20). Don't get lost in the "how" that we don't prepare for the promise.

Thought Question: What "how" has hindered you from experiencing the promises of God?

It's interesting to note that Zacharias was not offered an alternative or the opportunity to come out of the mute stage. God is just trying to bring us glad tidings and our natural being is literally blocking the supernatural move of God. As the old saints say, "Let God have His way."

(Luke 1:5-23) Zacharias was silenced until the birth of John because of his lack of faith. In the same chapter Mary, mother of Jesus and cousin of Elizabeth, goes to meet with her cousin to get some support from someone in a miraculous situation like hers. Mary was pregnant without having been with a man and Elizabeth was barren and too old, but God works in the impossible!

Therefore, no matter how old you are or how unprepared you may feel to bring forth all God has placed in you, trust me, you're chosen for such a time as this. (Isa 43:19 it is now time to bring forth)

Before we move on, let's study the sisterhood Elizabeth and Mary established in this chapter and how they handled their individual life altering experiences.

Luke 1: 24-25 NLT "Soon afterward his wife, Elizabeth, became pregnant and went into seclusion for five months. "How kind the Lord is!" she exclaimed. "He has taken away my disgrace of having no children."

The NLT makes Elizabeth's exclamation clear. Zacharias came back from his priestly duties and soon after Elizabeth became pregnant. The first point to notice is that supernatural things can happen in your life by being in the presence of God. I imagine the time in the temple that Zacharias had was a part of his normal routine as a priest and probably many times prayed for his wife to have children. However, this time there was a difference and he became speechless (Luke 1:23). Another great point is that there wasn't a long time from when the angel Gabriel delivered the word and Elizabeth became pregnant. Remember it doesn't take God a long time. The third point was that once Elizabeth confirmed she was pregnant she went into seclusion for five months. This would align the pregnancy in the second trimester, which is the best time to go public with your pregnancy especially if you've had complications in the past. Something to gain from this parallel is that not everyone needs to know just yet that you're pregnant. As the church mothers would say, "Hursh, and go sit down somewhere."

We must learn to just cover ourselves and the promise. The last point is how excited and grateful she was that the Lord had blessed her with a baby. Her reaction was totally different from her husbands'. The scripture never states that Zacharias tried to communicate what the angel said to him, but it implies that he and Elizabeth just went back to their normal lives after completion of his time at the temple. She may have wondered and probably was even scared to let anyone know, hence the seclusion, but either way she didn't doubt God.

I want to take a moment to elaborate on reasons for seclusion. Seclusion has gotten a bad rap for years, but there's a difference between being alone and loneliness. I suggest reading Dr. Myles Munroe's book "Single, Married, and Life after Divorce" for further explanation on understanding the difference.

Here are a few benefits of having alone time[2]

- Can improve concentration and memory
- Makes your interests a priority
- Boosts creativity
- Improves your relationships
- Makes you more productive
- Makes you more empathetic

Elizabeth took those five months, I assume, to focus on being in the best health for her and the baby, but possibly more as well. By the time Mary arrived, Elizabeth was confident that in spite of her natural obstacles she would begin her mom duties in just 3 months. This increased Mary's faith to not just believe the same could happen, but she stayed to see it come to pass (Luke 1:56).

God is sending some Mary's to some Elizabeth's. It's time to collaborate, encourage, motivate, be the example, and watch God increase your faith for the impossible. You may be reading this and saying I haven't met anyone that makes my baby leap. However, you will soon– stay alert. They may be closer than you think.

At six months, Mary came to visit Elizabeth because the angel Gabriel (Luke 1:36) told Mary that Elizabeth was pregnant, who was old and called barren. For with God all things are possible (Luke 1:37). This

---

[2] https://www.verywellmind.com/the-benefits-of-being-by-yourself-4769939

time when asked "how," the angel Gabriel did not recognize it as doubt but more of an inquiry. In turn, he explained how it was going to happen and even shared a testimony as encouragement to Mary that God is in control. We have to remember that God works in the impossible. Allow the testimonies of others to encourage you that what God has given you will come forth.

We will reference this story throughout this book because it aligns very well with a spiritual midwife. Even though the Bible doesn't go into details on what Mary did in those three months of her stay we can assume she helped around the home and learned from Elizabeth.

There's a blessing in having an "Elizabeth" in your life as a Mary and vice versa. Having a spiritual midwife is essential to bringing the child forth. In Biblical times there were only midwives that handled births, this was the norm. A midwife gives a trained professional opinion on what is best for you and the baby. A spiritual midwife prays and tarries with you until you are completely at peace. The Bible says our battle is through principalities and powers, so we can't just have a lot of good people around us but spiritually sound and anointed ones. Every good idea isn't a God idea.

Midwives are mentioned only six times in the Bible; and later on, we'll explain the importance of each mentioned. Now that we can see the necessity of a spiritual midwife, let's learn more about the "baby" in you.

HEART QUESTIONS: Who in your life can help you bring forth (list people by name here)? What are you actively doing to align yourself for these divine connections? What is holding you back (be honest)?

CHAPTER 3

Pregnant with Purpose

Finding out you are pregnant is one of the most exciting, nerve racking, and exuberant days of a woman's life. As a parent you begin to analyze everything you do, eat, drink, and even where you go. You become more concerned about what's in you. Some women are at their healthiest when they become pregnant, because it is no longer just about them.

The preparation is where many get stuck with sayings, "my blessings on the way", "the breakthrough is around the corner", and "it's coming." I'm sure if you've attended any church service once or twice you've heard this jargon before. I get it, the preacher or whomever is trying to encourage you to remain hopeful. However, when you find out you're pregnant with a baby you have an expected "due date."

Therefore, you honestly know the timeframe to expect this blessing to come forth. A spiritual midwife helps you during this process to do what's best for your body right before and as the changes begin to happen. As a spiritual midwife you'll have to remind the birther the best things needed to ensure their baby receives the best care within the womb. Many people have miscarried their purpose baby because they didn't have a midwife to guide them through the process.

Some may read this now and say yes that's all good Delisha, but I'm disciplined with my worship time, I'm studying, and spiritually/physically preparing for my "baby." Even the most disciplined athlete still needs the help of others to perform at her/his highest ability. Bringing forth what God has given does take discipline, but discipline is not the only thing you need in order to bring forth.

Points to focus on:

- Am I pregnant?

- Is it one or multiple babies?
- Finding your village
- Finding a spiritual midwife
- Preparing the environment
- 7 steps to prepare to nurture this child (place the foundation)

Am I pregnant?

Taking a pregnancy test to determine if you're pregnant is the first verification followed by a doctor's appointment. There's a difference between a feeling pregnant and actually being pregnant. The same is true in the spirit: we can often "feel" like something is our purpose or something we know God has promised us, but in reality it is something we've mesmerized so much that we just know it's God sent. I hate to be the bearer of bad news, but sweetie that's not God, that's a good idea.

Is it one or multiple babies?

The rarity of having twins is estimated that 1 in 250 natural pregnancies result in twins. So, it's not that uncommon that God may bless you with two promised babies to bring forth. Also, you may have more than one baby. I recall working with a mentor that explained to me that the two businesses they had were like their two babies and the best way to care for them was only by their leadership. Don't limit yourself to thinking that God can only use you to bring forth one amazing thing. He also may give you the grace to bring forth twins or more at the same time.

Once you have become clear on the number of babies you are currently pregnant with, it's time to focus on how you're going to prepare to bring the baby forth. Just as new parents prepare with reading, classes, and interviewing other parents with experience, the same is true for you. Begin to study those who have done things similar to you or better yet connect with those who are trendsetters. I believe we all have an original idea that no one else has. You are an original; and even if someone has a similar thing, you still have a God-given uniqueness. So make sure to seek the Creator for the best way to handle what He has given you.

Finding your village

This point can truly make a difference throughout and after the pregnancy. Having the right people around you is essential. As mentioned earlier, Elizabeth was in seclusion for five months, but in the six month her cousin Mary came to be with her until the baby came.

Two things to consider in building your village is:

- Is this the right time for this person?
- How can they be a support?

Don't just answer these questions yourself, but actually ask the person(s). It is important to communicate with the people you are bringing into your village. Communication helps overcome any possible future confusion or expectations. When everyone knows their role then they know how to be of the best support, or they can easily let you know maybe they can't help as they perceived earlier. Be prayerful and discern through the Spirit who is best for you at this time.

Finding a spiritual midwife

Pray about this and ask the Holy Spirit to lead you to this divine connection. Spiritual midwives often come into your life at the right time and aren't walking around with a shirt saying, "I'm your spiritual midwife." So it is essential to be very discerning on whom this may be. Also, keep in mind it may not be who you think it should be.

Aligning with your spiritual midwife has more to do with divine alignment than specific qualities. Marshawn Evans-Daniels defined:

supernatural alignment-- as being in position to hear, perceive, speak, receive and operate in the presence of God.

Therefore, being in alignment with the midwife for you begins with being aligned with God and headed in the right direction to what He has destined for you. I know there have been times in my life where I knew I wasn't alone in bringing forth a particular purpose God had for me and I needed the spiritual midwife more than I expected.

Preparing the environment

An area to not overlook is the environment you plan to nurture this baby. Even while writing this book, I've had to travel numerous times, so I had to write in environments that weren't ideal in order to complete this book. However, I was fortunate enough to be in seclusion in one of my close friend's home to complete the manuscript. The home was beautiful and peaceful to easily flush out everything God was downloading to me.

Thinking about the environment, I am reminded that Jesus' entrance into earth was at a manger in Bethlehem, which seemed opposite of where a future king would be born at. The environment needs to be the best place to securely bring forth all God has said with no complications. Jesus being born there kept him from being possibly found by King Herod's people, was a fulfillment of prophecy, and reflected His model of a servant-leader. Humbly entering the world and humbly becoming the redeemer of all mankind.

Growing up as a carpenter's son gave him no reputation until the appointed time of 30 to publicly go and display His true identity. From birth to Jesus' resurrection He was very specific about where He stayed, preached, performed miracles, prayed, and even who He let pray with Him. Our environment can influence our beliefs, values, thoughts, and behaviors. As you become more aligned with God, the more you'll see the impact an environment can have on you. Some of you may have to temporarily move away from your current environment.

I'd like to share some practical tips based on Biblical principles to discover your purpose before moving on to preparation for your purpose.

How to discover your God given purpose (tips from Dr. Myles Munroe)

1. Turn or Return to God-- Salvation is not about going to heaven, but rather we were saved to do work here on earth. (Your light must shine before people in such a way that they may see your good works, and glorify your Father who is in heaven. Matt. 5:16 NASB and "For we are his workmanship, created in Christ Jesus for good works, which God prepared beforehand, that we should walk in them." Eph 2:10 NASB) The uniqueness or secret about you is His glory (the true nature, full weight of something, the true essence of you is hidden in Him). The thing about you is that no one can "put their finger on it", "there's something about you", or "don't understand how you were able to be in a certain position, event, meeting, etc.". You've probably used one of these phrases before when entering places you may be even second guessing you belong. However, God is trying to show you

through these encounters that even if you can't see My glory on you others can.

2. <u>Ask yourself "What are my good works for which I was born?"</u> 1 Cor 2:1-16 (please read the entire chapter), verse 7 No, we declare God's wisdom, a mystery that has been hidden and that God destined for our glory before time began. There is secret wisdom hidden in God and the information is about two things; destiny and glory. The rulers of this age don't understand and the secret information isn't about Him but something He destined for you. The authorities of our culture can't give answers to why we exist. Don't trust anyone to tell you why you were born. Secret things are the thoughts of God that are found through the Spirit of God and the only thing to go deep in God to find out about you. (these things God has revealed to us through the Spirit. For the Spirit searches everything, even the depths of God. For who knows a person's thoughts except the spirit of that person, which is in him? So also no one comprehends the thoughts of God except the Spirit of God. 1 Cor. 2:10-11 ESV)

3. <u>No human can know the truth about you.</u> God kept the truth about you within Himself. No one knows the product like the Manufacturer. We keep manipulating life to figure out who we are and all we have to do is go to the Manufacturer. 1 Cor 2:11-13 (check Berean Study Bible)-- the only truth about you is in God. "the unbelievable truth, the truth about you will defy intellect, the truth about you will defy the assessment of others, the truth about you is beyond your knowledge and training, the truth about you can only be believed and received by your spirit first (your mind can't even believe it)."[examples

Abraham, Rahab, David, Moses,] No one can judge you when you become spiritually alive about who you are.

4. <u>Spend time with the Holy Spirit.</u> The key to the kingdom's secret about you is the Holy Spirit and why the whole world needs the Holy Spirit because without Him, what life are we living? Only the Spirit can tell the secret about you to you, the key to this whole thing is the Holy Spirit. The purpose of the Holy Spirit is to reveal the truth about ourselves, Are you living below your privilege? Please note: Awards can give you a false reality of who you really are. Just because we are good at something doesn't mean that's a part of our destiny. Remember good things aren't God things.

5. <u>5 points of the Holy Spirit</u> 1. No one can judge a spiritual man (1 Cor. 2:15) 2. Protects you from doing good things 3. The Holy Spirit gives you access to knowledge beyond your education (John 14:26 & 1 Cor 2:13) 4. The Holy Spirit gives you wisdom beyond your teachers (Ps 119:100) (how many people in the next ten years are you going to shock?) 5. The Holy Spirit gives you the understanding of principles with the ability to judge all things in life and spiritual things (1 Cor. 2:15-16). The kingdom of God is all about the Holy Spirit. Get the Holy Spirit and you will find your assignment.

Dr. Myles Munroe's mother once said "If you keep watching tv and not studying you'll die watching TV or you can be on it." Dr. Munroe is still being viewed by thousands of people around the world on TV, apps, and YouTube. To walk in your full assignment will require giving up something(s). Preparing for your "purpose baby" will require all of you (the glory of you) to be fully present in the process.

Now let's breakdown the Biblical examples: stories of Hannah and Sarah, who were two women that were barren that went on to have children that impacted nations.

7 steps to prepare to nurture the "promise" based on Hannah's life :

1. Pray consistently over the child (1 Sam 1:7 "So it was, year by year when she went up to the house of the LORD...")

2. Know how to respond with grace and surrender your all to God (1 Sam. 1:16 (ESV) Do not regard your servant as a worthless woman, for all along I have been speaking out of my great anxiety and vexation.")

3. Take your problems straight to God (1 Samuel 1:10 And she was in bitterness of soul, and prayed to the LORD and wept in anguish.)

4. Trust God to work on your behalf (1 Sam 1:11 Then she made a vow and said, "O LORD of hosts, if You will indeed look on the affliction of Your maidservant and remember me, and not forget Your maidservant, but will give Your maidservant a male child, then I will give him to the LORD all the days of his life, and no razor shall come upon his head.")

5. Believe that God will do what He said He'd do (1 Sam 1:18,20 And she said, "Let your maidservant find favor in your sight." So the woman went her way and ate, and her face was no longer sad. So it came to pass in the process of time that Hannah conceived and bore a son, and called his name Samuel, saying, "Because I have asked for him from the LORD.").

6. <u>Remain strong to uphold the faith in God's plan and sovereignty</u> (1 Sam. 1:24-28 Now when she had weaned him, she took him up with her, with three bulls, one ephah of flour, and a skin of wine, and brought him to the house of the Lord in Shiloh. And the child was young. 25 Then they slaughtered a bull, and brought the child to Eli. 26 And she said, "O my lord! As your soul lives, my lord, I am the woman who stood by you here, praying to the Lord. 27 For this child I prayed, and the Lord has granted me my petition which I asked of Him. 28 Therefore I also have lent him to the Lord; as long as he lives he shall be lent to the Lord." So they worshiped the Lord there.)

7. <u>Give God praise and remember God's faithfulness</u> (1 Sam 2:1-2 And Hannah prayed and said: "My heart rejoices in the Lord; My horn is exalted in the Lord. I smile at my enemies, Because I rejoice in Your salvation. "No one is holy like the Lord, For there is none besides You, Nor is there any rock like our God.)

*All above scripture references are NKJV unless indicated

God may not require of you to give what He promised completely back to Him. However, Hannah kept her word that she would give back to the Lord the very thing she had cried out years for. This story is very similar to that of Abraham in the willingness to sacrifice the very thing God promised.

Please note what you're believing Him for may be the exact thing He's asking you to surrender. Giving God your all is more than a cute saying or good phrase, but a true yes requires a sacrifice. Don't focus on losing something but gaining more. Hannah went on to give birth to five more children (1 Sam. 2:21). What you are about to birth may just be the beginning.

Another Bible story is Abraham and Sarah. You may have to relocate and disconnect from certain family members and friends to deliver what God has placed in you. Abraham and Sarah waited 25 years for the promise to be fulfilled, Issacs's birth.

5 takeaways from Abraham & Sarah on how to wait for that long promise:

1. Believe God the first time (Gen 12:3 NASB "...And in you all the families of the earth will be blessed.")

2. Don't try to help God bring the promise to fruition Abram and Sarai took the fulfillment of God's promise into their own hands. Abram appointed Elizer as the heir of his household (Gen. 15:3 But Abram said, "Lord GOD, what will You give me, since I am childless, and the]heir of my house is Eliezer of Damascus?). Sarai suggested Abram have a child with her handmaiden, Hagar (Gen 16:2-3 "So Sarai said to Abram, "See now, the LORD has prevented me from bearing children. Please have relations with my slave woman; perhaps I will obtain children through her." And Abram listened to the voice of Sarai. And so after Abram had lived ten years in the land of Canaan, Abram's wife Sarai took Hagar the Egyptian, her slave woman, and gave her to her husband Abram as his wife.").

3. Trust God when you don't know how it will get done. God still reassured them that the blessing will come through Abrams' loins. (Gen 15:4-8, "Then behold, the word of the LORD came to him, saying, "This man will not be your heir; but one who will come from your own body shall be your heir." And He took him outside and said, "Now look toward the heavens and count the stars, if you are able to count them." And He said to

him, "So shall your descendants be." Then he believed in the LORD; and He credited it to him as righteousness. And He said to him, "I am the LORD who brought you out of Ur of the Chaldeans, to give you this land to possess it."But he said, "Lord GOD, how may I know that I will possess it?")

4. God has an appointed time Gen 17; The Lord makes an official covenant with Abram and changes his name to Abraham and Sarai to Sarah. Abraham asked another question: will the fulfillment of this covenant/promise come through Ishmael and the Lord said no (v. 18). God gives the specific timeframe Sarah will give birth to Isaac (v. 21 But I will establish My covenant with Isaac, whom Sarah will bear to you at this season next year.").

5. Confirmation of the promise comes the closer you are Gen 18; Three men (that some commentators believe were angels) came to Abraham but only one speaks and says, "I will certainly return to you at this time next year; and behold, your wife Sarah will have a son (v. 10). Sarah, eavesdropping from the tent, laughed to herself, because she was now 90 and had been waiting 25 years on this "promise child." The Lord went to Abraham about Sarah laughing and said nothing is too hard for the Lord (v. 13 & 14 But the LORD said to Abraham, "Why did Sarah laugh, saying, 'Shall I actually give birth to a child, when I am so old?' Is anything too difficult for the LORD? At the appointed time I will return to you, at this time next year, and Sarah will have a son.").

The stories of Hannah and Sarah are that they both were barren women, but longed to have a child. They were both married to men of

God who had faith that one day they would. Another commonality is that they waited years for God to fulfill the promise.

Let me share a valuable tip, in this walk with God there is a lot of waiting.

Wait for the LORD;
Be strong and let your heart take courage;
Yes, wait for the LORD.
Psalm 27:14 NASB

A difference between the two women is that Hannah went on to have more children while Sarah had one physical child, but many in the faith. Both of the children went on to serve the Lord and lead the children of Israel. No matter if you have one baby or multiple, the impact that they will have on the world will be priceless. It's time to bring forth what God has destined specifically for you.

Now that we know a little more about what we're bringing forth, it's time to PUSH.

HEART QUESTIONS: How are you handling knowing your purpose? Are you taking steps daily to nurture your purpose? If not, why? What can you do today to change that?

CHAPTER 4

Push

Delivery is the most nervous, exciting, and often painful time of the entire process. The build up for this moment has been in preparation for an average time of nine months. The things the midwife has trained the birthers for is time to come to fruition and for the parents to implement what they've practiced so many times. We often have to push ourselves mentally as much as physically. The job of the midwife is to help the mother stay focused, relaxed, and keep a close watch on the health of the mother and baby.

It's time to push!

Your reason for picking up this book was just to get to this point. Everything around you is changing and the un-comfortableness is a sign it's time to bring forth. Like the people of Israel who were in such distress, that Hezekiah had to call for Isaiah the prophet to pray, because they had come this far but were unable to deliver. (They told him, "This is what Hezekiah says: This day is a day of distress and rebuke and disgrace, as when children come to the moment of birth and there is no strength to deliver them. Isaiah 37:3 NIV)

I want to take a break and speak this over your life and make this personal to say out loud:

1. I will deliver;
2. I have enough strength to deliver;
3. This is my time!

The time of "something is coming" or "on it's way" is over. Are you ready to "bring forth" is the question? Naturally, during the labor part– and especially the delivery, only a few people can be in the room once the baby is about to come forth.

The typical amount of people allowed in the delivery room is three. This number varies depending on the hospital and the severity of the delivering process. If many complications are happening the numbers may increase for hospital staff and just you. At no point will you ever be alone.

LABOR

You've come too far now to give up or lose strength. Previously mentioned in the labor process there are stages a woman experiences. A brief explanation and revelation of each stage is below.

Stage 1:

This is the longest stage with a two-part component of early and active labor. In early labor, contractions are irregular and mild. The length of this labor can last for hours and possibly days for first time mothers. On the other hand, active labor contractions are stronger, closer and regular. The average time of active labor is between 4-8 hours or longer. At this point the medical team may administer an epidural, if requested. The last part of active labor is the transition. During this time, contractions are close together and last up to 60-90 seconds. The mother now feels the urge to push and will feel pressure.

Stage one is an area we don't want prolonged. You may be reading this now and saying I'm in active labor and I have to get through this process to ensure my baby is delivered. Timing is key as it relates to labor and delivery. The question of the authenticity of this pregnancy is over, the real pain and pressure lies here. You have moved from early labor to active labor. This isn't like in the past where you thought something was going to happen or you got real close. It's time to bring forth!

Stage 2:

In stage two the mother will be asked to push during each contraction. During this stage the baby is moving through the birth canal. Once a baby is born, their airway is cleared (if need be) and the umbilical cord is cut. Right now everything is getting into alignment for your child to come forth. You are getting properly aligned with what you were purposed for.

Stage 3:

This is the shortest stage of labor; it can last from five minutes to an hour. The mother will still experience contractions and be asked to push one more time to deliver the placenta. Afterwards, the uterus continues to contract until it returns to its original size. Even though it's the shortest stage, it is the most vital to the mother's health. Retained placenta can cause unwanted side effects. Women's Integrated Healthcare says, "the delivery of the placenta represents the end of an important era living in the safety of your womb. It's the beginning of a new stage of life 'on the outside'."[3] You and your baby are entering a new stage of life, what nurtured the baby before is no longer of use. Behold, I am going to do something new, Now it will spring up; Isaiah 43:19a

Another complication that could happen during labor:

FTP stands for failure to progress and if this happens, various techniques, medicines and/or cesarean delivery is the only option to ensure the safety of mom and baby. If the extended period of time with progression continues the mother and baby both may be injured. Let's

---

[3] https://womensintegratedhealthcare.com/the-third-stage-of-labor-delivering-the-placenta/

go a little deeper into what these extended periods of time can look like for the mother and baby. The mother could have additional complications such as severe hemorrhaging, in which a hysterectomy is performed. A hysterectomy not only causes the mother the inability to bear children in the future, but also triggers premature menopause. Unpacking this in a spiritual sense, when you don't have the strength to push forth what God has given you and man's assistance/tools are used, the likelihood of having a safe delivery is jeopardized. We often say it's in God's hands but still rely on the plans of man alone. We are open to consequences of our actions not only endangering ourselves, but our baby and possible future babies. It's not enough to conceive the promise but we must also ask God to give us the ability to deliver full term what He has promised, with His strength. The promises God has placed in us are often impossible to man and therefore will take supernatural strength and great faith to bring forth. Which is why the next responsibility of the midwife is essential.

When to induce labor?

Inducing labor is not a common practice unless there is a true medical need for it. Healthcare providers want labor to take its natural course. However, in certain circumstances they will recommend inducing labor. Healthcare providers like to wait at least two weeks after the due date before inducing. I want to encourage someone who is thinking, "God, you said a year later, and that exact date was a week ago." Don't give up, because God is about to induce your labor.

DELIVERY

After the intensity of labor comes the beautiful delivery. The delivery is a sign you've not only carried a baby but you have toiled to bring it forth, and are now ready to nurture it to its full glory.

Whenever a woman is in labor she has pain, because her hour has come; but when she gives birth to the child, she no longer remembers the anguish because of the joy that a child has been born into the world. John 16:21

This joy may only last for a moment, but it's enough to get you through; and possibly cause you to decide to have more. However, the joy can fade after a few weeks as the nurturing in this new life begins to unfold.

The next chapter is important to prepare to read on what you have given up on that God has given you. Maybe there is something you've birthed, but don't feel qualified to take care of. Or maybe you feel like you have no help. This next chapter is for you.

HEART QUESTIONS: Why don't you want to push? Is it time to push? Who should be in the room when you push?

CHAPTER 5

Postpartum

The baby is here, now what?! This can be a very exciting and overwhelming time all at once; and sometimes not quite overwhelming until weeks or months later. I have a friend that I helped firsthand through this process. I drove 14 hours just to be there and assist her and her mom any way I could. Never being a mom myself nor having any medical background, I just did a quick search on postpartum before going on this impromptu trip. I went out of love for my sister-friend. I wanted her to know I was going to be right there even if it was just to drive, be in the room, change the baby, encourage her, etc.

This is often not just difficult for the mom, but also the baby because they've bonded with the mom for nine months and can sense emotional shifts. Also, if the mother has a spouse it can take a toil on him not knowing how to be a support. Postpartum depression doesn't happen to every mother, but it does happen enough for every mother to need to be prepared and have a plan in place on how to get through this phase.

Here are a few steps to help you get through this phase.

1. Seek help from someone who is trained in this area Ruth 3:6-8, 10-11, So she went down to the threshing floor and did according to all that her mother-in-law had commanded her. When Boaz had eaten and drunk and his heart was merry, he went to lie down at the end of the heap of grain; and she came secretly, and uncovered his feet and lay down. Then he said, "May you be blessed of the LORD, my daughter. You have shown your last kindness to be better than the first by not going after young men, whether poor or rich. "Now, my daughter, do not fear. I will do for you whatever you ask, for all my people in the city know that you are a woman of excellence. (Naomi

to Ruth); Esther 4:13-14, Then Mordecai told them to reply to Esther, "Do not imagine that you in the king's palace can escape any more than all the Jews. "For if you remain silent at this time, relief and deliverance will arise for the Jews from another place and you and your father's house will perish. And who knows whether you have not attained royalty for such a time as this?"(Mordecai to Esther).

2. Express your feelings with trusted friends and family members. Proverbs 17:17a, A friend loves at all times.

3. Join a support group of sisters/brothers that have experience with this. 1 Pet 5:9, (AMP) But resist him, be firm in your faith [against his attack--rooted, established, immovable], knowing that the same experiences of suffering are being experienced by your brothers and sisters throughout the world. [You do not suffer alone.]; Rom 8:17 and if children, heirs also, heirs of God and fellow heirs with Christ, if indeed we suffer with Him so that we may also be glorified with Him; Proverbs 27:17 Iron sharpens iron, So one man sharpens another; Hebrews 10:25 (NLT) And let us not neglect our meeting together, as some people do, but encourage one another, especially now that the day of his return is drawing near.

4. Find someone who can help take care of "the baby" (project, book, business, etc.) 1 Samuel 1:24-25, Now when she had weaned him, she took him up with her, with a three-year-old bull and one ephah of flour and a jug of wine, and brought him to the house of the LORD in Shiloh, although the child was young. Then they slaughtered the bull, and brought the boy to Eli.

5. <u>Rest as much as you can</u>-- try to get additional help so you can rest, Exodus 33:14, And He said, "My presence shall go with you, and I will give you rest."; Psalm 62:1-2 My soul waits in silence for God only; From Him is my salvation He only is my rock and my salvation, My stronghold; I shall not be greatly shaken; Psalm 116:7 Return to your rest, O my soul, For the LORD has dealt bountifully with you.

6. <u>Cut down on the least important responsibilities</u>-- use your time wisely, Phil 4:6-7, Be anxious for nothing, but in everything by prayer and supplication with thanksgiving, let your requests be made known to God. And the peace of God, which surpasses all comprehension, will guard your hearts and your minds in Christ Jesus; Ephesians 5:15-17 Therefore be careful how you walk, not as unwise men but as wise, making the most of your time, because the days are evil. So then do not be foolish, but understand what the will of the Lord is.

7. <u>Try not to worry about unimportant tasks</u>-- let me tell you what's unimportant: food, clothes, etc. Matt. 6:31-34, "So don't worry about these things, saying, 'What will we eat? What will we drink? What will we wear?' These things dominate the thoughts of unbelievers, but your heavenly Father already knows all your needs. Seek the Kingdom of God above all else, and live righteously, and he will give you everything you need. "So don't worry about tomorrow, for tomorrow will bring its own worries. Today's trouble is enough for today.

I interviewed a few mothers who had experience with postpartum depression or anxiety. Here are a few tips they shared:

1. This is nothing to be ashamed of and there is support. (Here's a link to find support today https://www.postpartum.net)
2. Don't be afraid to take a break. You're not the only one that can care for the baby.
3. No mother really knows what they're doing. You learn while on the job.

These tips are true after bringing forth what God has placed under your stewardship. After the tough work of delivering this baby, depression, anxiety, or distress may try to slip in. Sometimes one or all will, but don't let it limit you from being all that God has destined for you to be. The Psalmist David often lamented before the Lord from a depressed state he was in or anxiety he experienced while: running for his life from King Saul; his adulterous affairs; and enemies he faced. We all may experience some form of anxiety or depression, but we have hope in God so we don't stay there.

Mental health is a very important topic to me that definitely needs to be addressed within the Body of Christ. You can't just pray everything away. David often lamented before the Lord, but he made sure to give God praise more than complaining. Let your praise outweigh your frustration. David went on to write most of the longest books of the Bible, Psalms. David had more praises than laments.

Here are a few scriptures that will encourage you to truly lay your heart out before the Lord. Also, be encouraged that this anxiety or depression does not last forever.

"My soul [as well as my body] is greatly dismayed. But as for You, O LORD—how long [until You act on my behalf]?" Psalm 6:3 (AMP)

"Why do You stand afar off, O LORD? Why do You hide Yourself in times of trouble?" Psalm 10:1 (NASB)

"You have turned my mourning into joyful dancing. You have taken away my clothes of mourning and clothed me with joy, that I might sing praises to you and not be silent.

O LORD my God, I will give you thanks forever"! Psalm 30:11-12 (NLT)

"For our present troubles are small and won't last very long. Yet they produce for us a glory that vastly outweighs them and will last forever!" 2 Corinthians 4:17 (NLT)

Practical ways to handle PPD or anxiety[4]

- Don't face PPD alone—Seek help from a psychologist or other licensed mental health providers; contact your doctor or other primary health care provider. There's nothing to be ashamed of when experiencing PPD or anxiety.
- Talk openly about your feelings with your partner, other mothers, friends, and relatives.
- Join a support group for mothers—ask your health care provider for suggestions if you can't find one. (Heb 10:25)
- Find a relative or close friend who can help you take care of the baby. (Luke 1:26-40)
- Get as much sleep or rest as you can even if you have to ask for more help with the baby —if you can't rest even when you want to, tell your primary health care provider. (Ps. 62:1-2, 116:7)

---

[4] https://www.apa.org/pi/women/resources/reports/postpartum-depression

- As soon as your doctor or other primary health care provider says it's okay, take walks, get exercise. (Phil 4:13)
- Try not to worry about unimportant tasks—be realistic about what you can really do while taking care of a new baby. (Phil 4:6)
- Cut down on less important responsibilities (2 Cor 4:18)

Postpartum depression, anxiety, and distress are real, so make sure to assess some things you may be experiencing after bringing forth what God has given you. Later on we will discuss what a good steward looks like, but remember God will not put on you more than you can handle (1 Cor. 10:13). Your weakness is God's strength, He is mightier than anyone or anything.

"So I am well pleased with weaknesses, with insults, with distresses, with persecutions, and with difficulties, for the sake of Christ; for when I am weak [in human strength], then I am strong [truly able, truly powerful, truly drawing from God's strength]."

2 Cor. 12:10 (AMP)

HEART QUESTIONS: Are you experiencing postpartum anxiety or depression? (don't be ashamed if you are, you are not alone) Who can support you? (list their names and contact them today) If you have absolutely no one, email info@delishae.com. We'll connect you with resources and a free chat with me.

CHAPTER 6

Are you a Midwife?

The previous chapters have hopefully helped you answer these three questions:

1. What a midwife is?
2. Do you need one?
3. Are you one?

Midwives are not seeking the limelight and are often never recognized. The Bible only makes mention of midwives 9 times (Genesis 35:17, Genesis 38:28, and Exodus 1:15-21). One of the delays for me was truly being convicted of my calling, because I kept trying to compare something spiritual to a natural role/position or title. Oftentimes, especially as younger Believers, we try to make our calling make sense. God kept reminding me "I'm calling you a trendsetter so don't look for the blueprint you're making." Even with that Word from the Lord, I still for years was trying to make it make natural sense. As time went by and I became more mature within my purpose, I embraced what He'd been saying all along. I feel like Paul in Romans 4:21, "He was fully convinced that God is able to do whatever He promises." I don't need anyone to confirm what God has said.

Once I accepted the call of midwife and embraced what that looks like from a spiritual standpoint, I went to research everything I could find on a midwife. You probably thought I was going to say the Bible, but in 1 Corinthians 15:46 "The spiritual did not come first, but the natural, and after that the spiritual." There was so much information that made my spirit leap. It was like for the first time I was getting clarity on what I had done, was doing, and about to do. It also brought clarity as to why I was assigned to certain people and ministries to help bring something about, and once that was done the Lord directed me elsewhere.

Don't wait until someone prophesies to you: "I see you're called to be a midwife." Because, sweetheart, that day most likely will never come. It's not one of the nine gifts, so you may see yourself operating in numerous gifts but still feel God saying this role of midwife is for you. I believe the Holy Spirit teaches you all things (John 14:26) and, with that being said, I believe the Word of God (The Bible) has the explanations we need for life. In that same book of John, Jesus said the Holy Spirit will guide us (John 16:13). The Holy Spirit guided me through the scriptures and the midwife kept leaping out, so I began to study and receive clarity.

Responsibilities of a midwife:

- Examining (investigate thoroughly) and monitoring (check the progress or quality of something over a period of time; keep under systematic review) the pregnant women.
- Assessing (evaluate or estimate the nature, ability, or quality of) care requirements and writing care plans (a realistic customizable plan for the birther).
- Antenatal care (prenatal care) [reference who.int]
- Providing information, emotional support and reassurance to women and their partners (providing the scriptures specifically needed to process and deal with the changes happening to their family unit).
- Caring for and assisting women in labor (being right there to bring forth).
- Advising and supporting parents in the daily care of their newborn babies (ensuring the parents are thoroughly equipped and trained on how to care for that baby daily).
- Helping parents to cope with miscarriage, termination, stillbirth and neonatal death (The comfort and support needed

during this time is essential. Just because one promise wasn't fulfilled as we expected doesn't mean you want to have another and that you didn't grow from the experience.)

- Tutoring student midwives (pouring into the next generation of midwives.)
- Identifying high-risk pregnancies (a prophetic gift, visions and dreams on how to properly handle this specific pregnancy, the story of Rachel dying during the delivery of Benjamin (Genesis 35:18), she wanted to name him Ben-oni which means son of sorrow, but his father named him Benjamin which means, "son of my right hand")

The role of a midwife takes much discernment, because your level of involvement in one's life will change once "the baby" comes forth. Also, you may only be a midwife once for that person. Discernment is essential to maturing in your walk with God.

Discernment is simply the ability to judge well. As one matures in life, the decisions he or she makes will reflect the wisdom they have gained on this life's journey. We must be discerning of the times and what to do. 1 Chronicles 12:32 (NLT) states, "From the tribe of Issachar, there were 200 leaders of the tribe with their relatives. All these men understood the signs of the times and knew the best course for Israel to take."

Being aware of the times and knowing what to do is a gift from God. Only one tribe, Issachar, understood the signs of the times and the best course of action. We are living in a time of women rising up in leadership, especially women of color. However, what does that mean for women of God?:

1. Use this time to be aligned where God has assigned you;

2. Ask God to heighten your discernment on who to formulate your sisterhood with (Connect don't just network);

3. Bring every idea into reality because this is the time to shine. It is time to bring forth.

This book is not just for women however I am aware of the urgency that the Holy Spirit is placing on a lot of women's hearts that the time is NOW!

HEART QUESTIONS: Do you have a midwife? (remember they are there only for a season) Are you a midwife? If so, who should you be helping with their "baby" right now? (list their name and contact them)

_____

_____

_____

_____

_____

_____

_____

_____

_____

CHAPTER 7

Stay Connected to the Source

"Man can live 40 days without food, 3 days without water, 8 minutes without air, and 1 second without hope in God." – Anonymous

The easiest thing for a mature Believer to do is disconnect from God. Yes, you read that correctly. How? Simple we do it everyday, the more we memorize instead of treasure the Word of God (The Bible), the further away we are to Him. Unfortunately, "the church" has taught us to "praise our way through" in dance only or confess what someone has paraphrased at best what His Word says. However, the Bible says Jeremiah 1:12 (ESV), "Then the Lord said to me, "You have seen well, for I am watching over my word to perform it." The Lord watches over His word to perform it, not good sayings we have come up with and repeated. Now I believe in making positive confessions that align with scripture, but why not just confess the exact scripture. For example, pray like this According to 1 Peter 2:24, "...By Jesus Christ wounds I am healed." The same goes for praying for things to happen that may not be His will for our lives. The scripture says, "This is the confidence we have in approaching God: that if we ask anything according to His will, he hears us." (1 John 5:14). This scripture is often mis-interpreted because we just want to come before God asking for anything and totally forgetting the "His will" part.

Well, how do we know His will? First, we have to be connected to the Source. Without getting too deep in this part, the will of God is defined three ways in the Bible;

1. God's Sovereign Will (Eph. 1:11 & Acts 4:28);
2. God's Moral Will (Ex. 20:1-17);
3. God's Permissive Will (Acts 14:16).

Each of the wills of God is how the Holy Spirit directs us to pray concerning a matter and from there we can ask "anything." For example, if someone is dying and God's will is for them to transition from this world we can't pray for them to rise up, but we can pray for God to comfort the loved ones left behind and to give them peace in the coming days.

Staying connected to God is hard because it's so easy to disconnect from Him. The more we play "church", memorize cliches, attend prayerless services and make fasting rituals, and simply stop reading His Word, the further apart we are from Him. Sometimes we equate how long we've been a Believer to a level of maturity we realistically have not achieved. There's a difference between knowing God and knowing of God. For example, I know of Lebron James but I don't know Lebron James. That small preposition "of" makes a world of difference. Matthew 7:23 (NKJV), "And then I will declare to them, 'I never knew you; depart from Me, you who practice lawlessness!" I don't know about you, but I want God to "know" me when I arrive at heaven's gates.

The same way you became to know of God when you first believe is the same way you must stay connected with Him as you live this life. Like any relationship if you BOTH don't make the effort to communicate, spend time together, and love each other it won't last. Let this not be said of us, "Yet I hold this against you: You have forsaken the love you had at first." (Revelation 2:4 NIV). I want to keep that same love I had for God from the beginning. NEVER lose that! Some say, "As you mature you don't do all that running, jumping, and telling everybody you know about Jesus." However, I've found that when I'm not telling someone about God I'm often getting far from Him myself.

Who have you testified about the goodness of God to this month? Exactly! When we first get engaged, we tell everyone without them asking. We find a way to bring it up in conversation. The same is true for God, Jesus and the Holy Spirit. Bring them up in conversation on purpose. I used to be hesitant to say the Spirit revealed to me "xyz" and that's how I know to those who weren't Believers. I found myself stuttering and not able to articulate what I knew. Sometimes the more we "know" the less we know God. Don't let your intellect disconnect you from God.

Trying to always align the natural with the spirit will cause you to be confused and sometimes even doubt what you believe. The premise of Christianity, if you will, is faith. I don't argue with people over things like the color of Jesus' skin, pre- or post-tribulation, and a list of other things, because the bottom-line is established on faith. That's why I often advise people who are trying to understand God and new Believers to read the Bible for themselves. The Bible is the written Word of God. How much more can you come to believe in Him unless learning more about Him?

Taking time away from what distracts YOU is essential to ensuring you stay connected with God. It's known that most churches do a congregational fast in the month of January, which may include increased prayer time, limited foods (vegetarian diet), no media or limited, and no sugars. However, what happens by February... People indulge back where they left off or pick up completely new habits. I'm not a big sweets person and I have a plant-based diet, so for me nothing major changed. However, where I gained the most revelation was the purposeful time spent praying and reading the Bible.

Fun fact, according to Dr. Caroline Leaf, "it takes a minimum of 63 days to change an automated habit..." With that fact, imagine how much time we need to spend just changing one automated habit we have. This is also one more reason why we need the help of God to do anything. We must stay connected.

WAYS TO STAY CONNECTED:

1. Talk to God daily;
2. Fast often;
3. Create a realistic schedule to do 1 and 2;
4. Get an accountability partner.

HEART QUESTIONS: How are you staying connected to God? What is hindering you from connecting? Do you need accountability in this area?

CHAPTER 8

The Due Date

I thought that Chapter 7 was all God could give me to share, but there's more. The significance of the number eight speaks volumes to the season you are entering, new beginnings. You are not only bringing forth the fruit within, but this won't be like any other "pregnancy." Remember cramps don't mean you are in labor, just like passion doesn't equal purpose. However, you are entering the season where there will be no more false alarms. This is the real thing.

For some of you, the fruit within has been lying dormant, but now the urgency to write that book, launch that business, go back to school, make that investment, and love that family member is now. Being intentional for the next 60 days on where you are going in the next six months allows you to build habits that can get you there when you don't "feel like it." From the conception of this book to delivery it wasn't an easy process; and many times I wanted to postpone the due date, because of life. A baby doesn't stop going through the delivery process just because it's an inconvenience to the parents.

After having a conversation with a fellow author, he resonated with simply the title of this book and said I need to really finish my book immediately. Today you picked up this book for numerous reasons, but I'd venture to say you are ready to bring forth everything God has destined for you to do.

Don't forget to nurture that baby

Real parenting begins after the baby comes and is why midwives help the parents establish a new schedule to their newfound way of life. Nurturing includes: the care for; encouraging the development of; and the cherishing of the God-given promise. You don't care for something you cherish the same way you do for things that you don't really value.

Cherish- protect and care for (someone) lovingly, hold (something) dear, keep (a hope or ambition) in one's mind.

Handling your gifts with a spirit of excellence quickly gets you to the place God has given you. The way you handle the gifts in a spirit of excellence will get you far with what God has given you. This is not the time to haphazardly commit to this new lifestyle, but rather lean all the way into it. Begin associating yourself with like-minded individuals who are further along, as well as some on a similar journey to have that support system. Support can get you further than solo skills. The age old saying, "It's not about what you know, but who you know." This has held to be true in my life and others. So, before you bring forth, make sure to build that village to help nurture this "baby."

Here are a few tips:

<u>Let it grow</u>

Starting a business or becoming an author is easier said than done, because most of the work isn't glamorous. However, from the very beginning, always prepare to scale. You may not have everything you need now but you can see the future of this so plan for that reality. Right now you may be in a storefront, but you see the store in malls around the world. One mentor told me, "The difference between those who want to be authors and those who are is one word, execution." Today take a step towards the preparation for growth. First expand your thinking, secondly stretch your faith, and lastly accept that God knows the details. These last days we need GREAT faith to fulfill all that God has destined for our lives. "Do not despise these small beginnings, for the LORD rejoices to see the work begin..." Zechariah 4:10 NLT

<u>Keep checking in</u>

Just how your children in the natural world will always be your babies no matter how old they are, it is the same thing you're purposefully bringing forth. After that business has reached a level, someone else can manage the day-to-day and run with the vision, however, it's always good to still check in. Checking in helps keep the vision aligned with an ever evolving mission of the organization.

In the world we live in, everyone is taught to be a "boss", but God told us to be good stewards and follow the example of Jesus in servant-leadership form. Someone once described the kingdom of God as the "opposite kingdom" because everything the scriptures share on behaviors and characteristics are often opposite of society. So what's the difference between a steward and a boss?

Steward	Boss
One who manages, supervises; one who actively direct affairs; fiscal agent (a person who likes after passengers on a ship); one employed in a large household or estate to manage domestic concerns	A person who exercises control or authority.
Focuses on taking care of their team, product, and customers.	Focuses on controlling people.

The term steward is recognized as someone taking the responsibility of managing others.	The saying "Boss" generally isn't in power, but is someone trying to express a kind of power.
Character examples: Khadijah James (Living Single), Lorelai Gilmore (Gilmore Girls), Leslie Knope (Parks and Recreation)	Character examples: Mr. Burns (The Simpsons), Wilhelmina Slater (Ugly Betty), Miranda Priestly (The Devil Wears Prada), Buddy Ackerman (Swimming with Sharks)
Origination: Old English word dating back to the early 17th century to describe one who has the superintendence of household affairs, guardian.	Origination: Dutch in origin and another word to describe a "master" in slavery back in 1806.

Do you still want to be addressed as a "boss"? Don't let this world distract you from your purpose of being here, you are just a sojourner passing through (Beloved, I beseech you as sojourners and pilgrims, to abstain from fleshly lusts, which war against the soul; 1 Peter 2:11 ESV)

My prayer for you is that you will not only bring forth this "baby," but continue to birth what's in you. We need all of you to come forth now. Whenever you're reading this the time is, NOW! You haven't read this far just to say, "that was a good read" without any action plans to change the current story of your legacy. Before I close with an actual confession let me say, do not compare your portion with others. In 1

Corinthians 12 it breaks down the need of every person in the Body of Christ. Don't try to be the head when your role is the big toe. You pursuing something that's not for you causes the entire body to limp. For years I did certain things just because I could and was good at them. However, being good at something doesn't mean you're called to do that. Yep, read that again.

Don't let your skills limit you from your calling. We can be multifaceted, but usually there are always one or two things that wake us up early and make us stay up late. The things you would do without getting paid are often aligned with your divine assignment, because usually it is closely aligned with your characteristics.

Fruit versus Gift

Writing this chapter I changed the reference of the "baby" from gift to fruit, because fruit is a production of the root, it has the same DNA. While a gift is something one can obtain but easily lose, give away, or worse, destroy. The fruit of you is about to be brought forth. This fruit is a reflection of YOU, remember that as more people want access to the baby.

Due Date CONFESSION

My time is now!

It is time for me to accept what I was created for.

Thank you God for divine alignment with those who will help me on this journey.

Thank you God for continued discernment on relationships, partnerships, and business endeavors.

My time is now and this is only the beginning.

God, increase my faith to not only believe, but to execute on all you've given me.

My time is Now!

The LORD will fulfill his purpose for me; your steadfast love, O LORD, endures forever. Do not forsake the work of your hands. Psalm 138:8 ESV

HEART QUESTIONS: Have you come to the realization that the time is now? If so, write the vision here. Give yourself a realistic date to bring this purposeful fruit to earth. What do you need to do? (make a list and get to work)

This poem was written by my beloved Auntie Nadine Howard, I will always love you and thank you for your words. I commit to share them with the world!

TIME

Time is limitless;
it waits for no one, use yours wisely.
If you're not watchful of it;
It will leave before you get started
God is everything; time is within Him
He doesn't operate on our time,
only through the time He's given us.
We don't realize His timing is perfect,
until our set time has passed.
We think He's forgotten about us
But His time for that moment has just begun
to unfold into a lifetime of
possibilities only He can give.

-Nadine Howard

JOURNAL SECTION

Made in the USA
Middletown, DE
11 March 2022

62407018R00055